SELECTING MEGAVOLTAGE
TREATMENT TECHNOLOGIES
IN EXTERNAL BEAM RADIOTHERAPY

The following States are Members of the International Atomic Energy Agency:

AFGHANISTAN
ALBANIA
ALGERIA
ANGOLA
ANTIGUA AND BARBUDA
ARGENTINA
ARMENIA
AUSTRALIA
AUSTRIA
AZERBAIJAN
BAHAMAS
BAHRAIN
BANGLADESH
BARBADOS
BELARUS
BELGIUM
BELIZE
BENIN
BOLIVIA, PLURINATIONAL
   STATE OF
BOSNIA AND HERZEGOVINA
BOTSWANA
BRAZIL
BRUNEI DARUSSALAM
BULGARIA
BURKINA FASO
BURUNDI
CAMBODIA
CAMEROON
CANADA
CENTRAL AFRICAN
   REPUBLIC
CHAD
CHILE
CHINA
COLOMBIA
COMOROS
CONGO
COSTA RICA
CÔTE D'IVOIRE
CROATIA
CUBA
CYPRUS
CZECH REPUBLIC
DEMOCRATIC REPUBLIC
   OF THE CONGO
DENMARK
DJIBOUTI
DOMINICA
DOMINICAN REPUBLIC
ECUADOR
EGYPT
EL SALVADOR
ERITREA
ESTONIA
ESWATINI
ETHIOPIA
FIJI
FINLAND
FRANCE
GABON

GEORGIA
GERMANY
GHANA
GREECE
GRENADA
GUATEMALA
GUYANA
HAITI
HOLY SEE
HONDURAS
HUNGARY
ICELAND
INDIA
INDONESIA
IRAN, ISLAMIC REPUBLIC OF
IRAQ
IRELAND
ISRAEL
ITALY
JAMAICA
JAPAN
JORDAN
KAZAKHSTAN
KENYA
KOREA, REPUBLIC OF
KUWAIT
KYRGYZSTAN
LAO PEOPLE'S DEMOCRATIC
   REPUBLIC
LATVIA
LEBANON
LESOTHO
LIBERIA
LIBYA
LIECHTENSTEIN
LITHUANIA
LUXEMBOURG
MADAGASCAR
MALAWI
MALAYSIA
MALI
MALTA
MARSHALL ISLANDS
MAURITANIA
MAURITIUS
MEXICO
MONACO
MONGOLIA
MONTENEGRO
MOROCCO
MOZAMBIQUE
MYANMAR
NAMIBIA
NEPAL
NETHERLANDS
NEW ZEALAND
NICARAGUA
NIGER
NIGERIA
NORTH MACEDONIA
NORWAY

OMAN
PAKISTAN
PALAU
PANAMA
PAPUA NEW GUINEA
PARAGUAY
PERU
PHILIPPINES
POLAND
PORTUGAL
QATAR
REPUBLIC OF MOLDOVA
ROMANIA
RUSSIAN FEDERATION
RWANDA
SAINT LUCIA
SAINT VINCENT AND
   THE GRENADINES
SAMOA
SAN MARINO
SAUDI ARABIA
SENEGAL
SERBIA
SEYCHELLES
SIERRA LEONE
SINGAPORE
SLOVAKIA
SLOVENIA
SOUTH AFRICA
SPAIN
SRI LANKA
SUDAN
SWEDEN
SWITZERLAND
SYRIAN ARAB REPUBLIC
TAJIKISTAN
THAILAND
TOGO
TRINIDAD AND TOBAGO
TUNISIA
TURKEY
TURKMENISTAN
UGANDA
UKRAINE
UNITED ARAB EMIRATES
UNITED KINGDOM OF
   GREAT BRITAIN AND
   NORTHERN IRELAND
UNITED REPUBLIC
   OF TANZANIA
UNITED STATES OF AMERICA
URUGUAY
UZBEKISTAN
VANUATU
VENEZUELA, BOLIVARIAN
   REPUBLIC OF
VIET NAM
YEMEN
ZAMBIA
ZIMBABWE

The Agency's Statute was approved on 23 October 1956 by the Conference on the Statute of the IAEA held at United Nations Headquarters, New York; it entered into force on 29 July 1957. The Headquarters of the Agency are situated in Vienna. Its principal objective is "to accelerate and enlarge the contribution of atomic energy to peace, health and prosperity throughout the world".

IAEA HUMAN HEALTH REPORTS No. 17

SELECTING MEGAVOLTAGE TREATMENT TECHNOLOGIES IN EXTERNAL BEAM RADIOTHERAPY

INTERNATIONAL ATOMIC ENERGY AGENCY
VIENNA, 2022

COPYRIGHT NOTICE

© IAEA, 2022

Printed by the IAEA in Austria
January 2022
STI/PUB/1948

IAEA Library Cataloguing in Publication Data

Names: International Atomic Energy Agency.
Title: Selecting megavoltage treatment technologies in external beam radiotherapy / International Atomic Energy Agency.
Description: Vienna : International Atomic Energy Agency, 2022. | Series: IAEA human health reports, ISSN 2074–7667 ; no. 17 | Includes bibliographical references.
Identifiers: IAEAL 21-01424 | ISBN 978–92–0–116821–4 (paperback : alk. paper) | ISBN 978–92–0–116921–1 (pdf) | ISBN 978–92–0–117021–7 (epub)
Subjects: LCSH: Cancer — Radiotherapy. | Radiotherapy, High Energy. | Medical physics.
Classification: UDC 615.849 | STI/PUB/1948

FOREWORD

The global incidence of cancer is rising significantly, with low and middle income countries (LMICs) experiencing the highest increases. Radiotherapy is one of the three main modalities for the treatment of cancer, along with surgery and chemotherapy. The aim of radiotherapy is to control a malignant tumour by exposing it to a high dose of radiation, while at the same time limiting to acceptable levels the radiation dose received by normal tissue. In the light of the rising cancer incidence and the lack of sufficient treatment capabilities, the need for additional radiation treatment technologies is considerable. This is particularly the case in LMICs, where the shortage of radiotherapy capabilities is acute. In preparation for the expected increases in cancer incidence and in the corresponding number of patients in the coming decade, a large number of new high energy radiotherapy machines capable of delivering megavoltage beams will be required globally. However, the answer is not simply to buy a new linear accelerator (linac) or ^{60}Co teletherapy machine.

Radiotherapy can be delivered with different types of machine, such as external beam high energy radiation machines, kilovoltage machines and brachytherapy equipment. Variations in the incidence of different cancer types, the complexity and cost of treatment technologies, and differences in local social, economic and physical circumstances are all factors that influence technology acquisition, purchase and implementation.

The radiotherapy treatment process is itself complicated and involves much more than just radiotherapy machines. A cancer diagnosis requires, at a minimum, pathology and diagnostic imaging. Once radiotherapy is prescribed, imaging is needed to determine the location and extent of the disease. Without adequate numbers of professionally trained radiation oncologists, medical physicists and radiation therapists, treatment cannot proceed accurately or safely.

This publication addresses just one of the many factors, albeit an important one, associated with the planning of a new radiotherapy facility or the upgrade of an existing one. This concerns the selection of a high energy (megavoltage) radiotherapy machine. The two main high energy machine types are linacs and ^{60}Co machines. Although both treatment modalities have been compared extensively in the relevant literature, very few publications describe all the issues to consider when choosing a megavoltage machine. This publication puts all appropriate questions into context and provides information for non-technical administrators and decision makers, and for professionals directly involved in treating patients.

The IAEA wishes to express its gratitude to the authors and reviewers of this publication, in particular J. Van Dyk (Canada). The IAEA officer responsible for this publication was K. Christaki of the Division of Human Health.

CONTENTS

1. INTRODUCTION

1.1. BACKGROUND

Radiotherapy is one of the major treatment modalities for cancer, along with surgery and chemotherapy. It has been shown to be cost effective in many countries, including in low and middle income countries (LMICs) [1, 2]. Depending on the predominance of specific cancers in the geographic region in question, approximately 40–60% of all cancer patients can benefit from radiotherapy [3–6]. The process of radiotherapy is complex, involving multiple steps, multiple technologies and many different professional staff, as indicated in Appendix I. Radiotherapy involves technologies that go well beyond radiation treatment machines alone. Furthermore, numerous professionals with different expertise are involved in the process.

In terms of the actual radiation dose delivery, external beam radiotherapy most commonly uses megavoltage photons from linear accelerators, also known as linacs, or from ^{60}Co machines. In principle, the term 'megavoltage' refers to the accelerating potential of the electrons striking the target of a linac and is conventionally used as an X ray quality specifier. However, since the average energy of a linac is of the same order of magnitude as the average photon energy of a ^{60}Co beam (i.e. 1.25 MeV), the terms 'megavoltage beams', 'photons' or 'radiation' are also commonly used to describe the quality of ^{60}Co radiation, no matter how the radiation is generated.

There has been much discussion in the literature about the advantages and disadvantages of one delivery machine over another [3–17]. The decision making process regarding which technology to implement is complex, since the considerations are multifactorial, relating not only to the patients, the availability of professional staff and the technical issues associated with each technology, but also to cost considerations, radiation safety and security issues, and the need for, and availability of, local servicing and maintenance. Regarding safety, it is important, for instance, to consider that the radiation from a ^{60}Co source cannot be 'turned off'. Such sources need continual shielding and other radiation protection measures, and their safety needs to be managed during their entire lifespan. On the other hand, maintenance is much less demanding for ^{60}Co machines, since the underlying technology is less advanced than that of linacs.

Figure 1 illustrates that approximately 25% of the IAEA–WHO dosimetry audits conducted in 2013 were for ^{60}Co beams, and suggests that the utilization of linac beams is increasing overall. In 2019, approximately 3485 linacs and 1746 ^{60}Co machines were in clinical service in LMICs [18]. In Africa, if countries with established radiotherapy services such as South Africa, Morocco, Algeria and Egypt are removed from the statistics, ^{60}Co based radiotherapy units constituted approximately 33% of the number of treatment units installed in the region in 2019 [18]. In terms of future projections, a 2015 Lancet Oncology Commission report [1] estimated that by 2035 an additional 8400 machines will be required in LMICs to ensure an availability of radiotherapy that is equal in all income environments.

1.2. OBJECTIVE

While sustainability is difficult to predict and uncertainties in the numerical values of these equipment related projections may exist, the message is clear: there is an enormous need for more radiation treatment machines throughout the world. The objective of this publication is to address which type of technology to implement, and to determine the issues surrounding appropriate decisions in consideration of the multiple variables associated with new machine acquisition.

This publication is primarily aimed at the key individuals involved in the decision making process regarding technology purchase and implementation of radiotherapy, such as upper level managers, administrators, the heads of radiation oncology and medical physics departments.

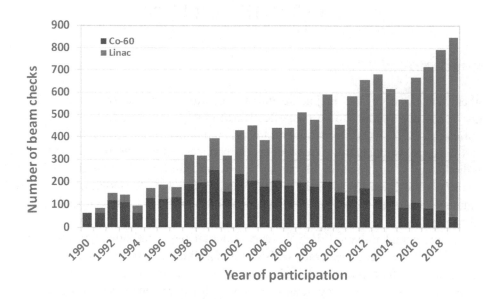

FIG. 1. *The number of* ^{60}*Co and linac beams checked using the IAEA–WHO reference beam dosimetry audit service per year.*

Guidance provided here, describing good practices, represents expert opinion but does not constitute recommendations made on the basis of a consensus of Member States.

1.3. SCOPE

This publication does not provide a simple answer as to whether ^{60}Co machines, standard single energy linacs or complex multienergy linacs should be chosen in the technology acquisition process. Rather, the scope of this publication is to provide information such that each decision making group will be able to ask the appropriate questions to allow informed decisions to be made locally, taking into consideration existing infrastructure and resources. The emphasis is on the purchase of ^{60}Co machines, standard single energy linacs or complex multienergy linacs.

Standard single energy linacs are considered to be single energy machines that have a flattening filter and no kilovoltage imaging (i.e. they are not complex, advanced or specialized single energy machines such as CyberKnife, TomoTherapy, Gamma Knife or Halcyon systems). A complex multienergy machine, on the other hand, can provide more than one photon energy, a choice of electron energies, and include kilovoltage or megavoltage imaging.

More advanced technologies such as helical tomotherapy, robotic radiotherapy or treatments using heavier particles (such as protons and carbon ions) are not considered in this publication.

1.4. STRUCTURE

Section 2 provides an overview of a typical national cancer control planning process. Section 3 describes a typical equipment selection and customization process. Section 4 lays out the clinical factors that influence technology acquisition, and Section 5 looks at the main technical characteristics of ^{60}Co teletherapy machines and linacs. Section 6 provides a discussion on the infrastructure and maintenance requirements. Section 7 lists the main essential components currently available beyond the treatment machines, and Section 8 provides cost estimates for the facility and its construction and maintenance, and for equipment including operating costs, and personnel. Section 9 concludes with a detailed summary and comparison of ^{60}Co teletherapy machines and linacs.

Appendix I describes the steps involved in the typical radiation treatment process, including the technologies used at each stage and the professional staff typically involved. Appendix II contains a series of questions for consideration as part of the technology acquisition process, and Appendix III gives information on the standard equipment package required for a radiotherapy department. Appendices IV and V address how to calculate the number of machines required.

2. NATIONAL CANCER CONTROL PLANNING

Radiotherapy services in the public sector are normally centrally planned and managed by the national health authority. A strategic task force committee ideally performs an ongoing review to monitor indications as to whether additional treatment capabilities need to be acquired. Various publications addressing in detail these indications have been developed by the IAEA [15] and others [19, 20].

National healthcare planners who are preparing for the implementation of radiotherapy services, including the purchase of technologies that are appropriate for and compatible with country-specific needs and conditions, may consider the following:

(a) Disease types (based on data from the national cancer registry, or, if one does not exist, based on data estimated by GLOBOCAN [21]);
(b) Patient numbers (based on data from population censuses and statistics on distribution of age and gender);
(c) Distribution of the population in the country;
(d) Financial model and funding allocation for healthcare;
(e) Personnel status, including numbers, professional knowledge, competence and training and education requirements;
(f) Local environmental conditions, including reliability of electrical supply and ability to control humidity and temperature in the treatment and equipment rooms;
(g) Connectivity of radiotherapy equipment within service clusters (e.g. treatment delivery machines, simulators, treatment planning computers, quality control equipment, dosimetry equipment, treatment record, verification system/computer network);
(h) Availability of supporting clinical services (e.g. diagnostic imaging, surgery, chemotherapy, laboratory services, hospital information systems);
(i) Sustainability, as regards availability of local expertise (e.g. structural, information technology (IT), logistics, finance), availability of replacement parts, availability of maintenance service contracts.

Many of these issues are addressed in more detail in subsequent sections of this publication.

3. EQUIPMENT SELECTION AND CUSTOMIZATION PROCESS

3.1. CORE IMPLEMENTATION TEAM

Once a decision has been made to procure new radiotherapy machines, it is recommended that a second professional team, called the core implementation team, is established to manage the project [22]. Reference [22] gives the following advice on building a core implementation team.

"At a minimum, the team should consist of the following:

— A qualified architect, preferably experienced in the design and construction of radiation oncology facilities.
— A structural or civil engineer with experience in large concrete structures (e.g. dams or other large concrete structures). Expertise in casting large volumes of concrete is a requirement.
— A mechanical engineer with experience in hospital design, including cooling, heating and ventilation systems.
— An electrical engineer experienced in the calculation and design of reticulation and standby electrical systems for hospitals. The ability to design the information technology (IT) and communication reticulation is highly recommended.
— A cost consultant or quantity surveyor or equivalent.
— A clinically qualified radiotherapy medical physicist with competency in the planning of new departments in similar environments. It is important that the medical physicist can participate fully in the specification and commissioning of appropriate equipment in order to provide the maximum possible access to radiotherapy, taking into consideration the prevailing infrastructure and resource constraints.
— A qualified radiation oncologist experienced in setting up and coordinating a radiation oncology facility within a system of similar resources is highly recommended.

"In all cases where the expertise is not locally available and an external expert is recruited to assist, a local consultant should be designated for shadowing purposes."

Additional advisers can be made part of the team or brought in on an as-needed basis, such as in the case of IT and machine servicing support. This team needs to be in close communication with the regulatory agency involved in licensing the facility, as well as with the vendor, once a specific machine to be purchased has been selected. The findings of the team are to be reported to the strategic task force. In this publication, it is assumed that a national cancer control plan exists [17], that a local needs assessment has been performed [15, 19] and that a decision has been made to purchase megavoltage radiotherapy technologies (whether ^{60}Co machine(s), linac(s) or both).

3.2. SELF-ASSESSMENT QUESTIONNAIRE

Throughout this publication, various questions are posed that need to be answered by the strategic task group and core implementation team. These can be used in the planning and implementation process. These questions form a self-assessment questionnaire that is given in Appendix II.

4. CLINICAL FACTORS IN TECHNOLOGY ACQUISITION

From a radiobiological perspective, gamma rays from ^{60}Co machines have the same linear energy transfer and, therefore, the same radiobiological response as X rays from high energy linacs [23]. From a clinical perspective, only a few trials have compared ^{60}Co gamma rays and high energy X rays. A review by Urtasun [24] in 1992 reported that improvement in therapeutic results was made possible by advances in the physical delivery of radiation from the older medium energy kilovoltage machines (200–400 kV) to megavoltage treatment machines that included ^{60}Co and linacs. Furthermore, with computed tomography (CT) simulation and three dimensional (3-D) treatment planning systems, it was possible to shape fields and design beams to individualize patient treatments much more confidently. One clinical study comparing 6 MV with 4 MV photons and ^{60}Co found no difference in tumour control for glottic cancer [25]. Another study made a direct comparison between ^{60}Co and 6 MV irradiation for over 1450 head and neck cancer cases [26]. The study found that 6 MV was equivalent to ^{60}Co, except possibly for postoperative patients at high risk of neck relapse, for whom ^{60}Co seemed to provide better control to the neck nodes than 6 MV. This was largely due to the higher surface dose from the shallower buildup depth for ^{60}Co. Superior dose distributions could be obtained with ^{60}Co for advanced disease extending to the surface (e.g. an exenterated orbital tumour with positive margins).

The dose to bone increases with an increase in lower energy photons owing to the physical interaction mechanism. Large ^{60}Co fields have a significantly lower energy scatter component, such as those used for half-body irradiation or total body irradiation. Cobalt-60 gives a 4% higher dose to bone compared with 6 MV and a 10% higher dose to bone compared with 18 MV [27, 28]. For smaller field sizes, these differences are significantly smaller. If total body irradiation is used for bone marrow transplants, the higher dose to bone could be considered by some to be an advantage. It might also be an advantage when using large fields (e.g. half-body irradiation) for the treatment of bone metastases [29].

5. TECHNICAL COMPARISON BETWEEN ^{60}Co TELETHERAPY MACHINES AND LINACS

Various groups have published a technical comparison between ^{60}Co teletherapy machines and linacs [3, 11, 12, 15, 16, 19]. An overview is given in this section and the main criteria for comparison are summarized in Table 1 (which is adapted from table 1 of Ref. [16]).

5.1. BEAM ENERGY CONSIDERATIONS

Regarding the choice of beam energy, various opinions have been published [4, 12, 30–34]. Laughlin et al. [31] argue for the advantages of 4–8 MV photons versus ^{60}Co. However, Suit [4] maintains that there is still a major role for ^{60}Co. Similarly, Van Dyk and Battista [16] contend that given the optimum circumstances of various energies being available, about 25% of radical cases could benefit from ^{60}Co teletherapy with conventional treatment approaches.

Among the multiple perspectives found in the literature, several considerations are recognized. For instance, currently 6 MV is the commonest choice of energy for single energy standard linacs, as well as for helical tomotherapy and robotic radiotherapy. However, if electron beam therapy is desired, most standard machines with this option also offer additional higher photon beam energies.

TABLE 1. CRITERIA TO CONSIDER WHEN IMPLEMENTING NEW RADIATION TREATMENT TECHNOLOGIES [16][a]

Criteria	Considerations
Clinical	Estimated number of curative patients
	Estimated number of palliative patients
	Disease sites to be treated
	Stage of the disease
Radiation beam characteristics	Beam edge sharpness
	Beam penetration/buildup (energy)
	Scattering conditions/dose uniformity
	Contour/inhomogeneity corrections
	Dose to bone
Machine characteristics	Dose rate
	Patient to collimator distance
	Radioactive source versus X rays
	Multiple photon energies
	Electron beams
Technique options	2-D, 3-D, 4-D
	Beam shaping/multileaf collimation
	IMRT[b]/VMAT[c] capable
	IGRT[d] capable
	High dose rate mode
Infrastructure/service/maintenance issues	Local services (water, electricity, transportation) Room and shielding requirements
	Machine service availability
Safety considerations	Radiation protection Security of radioactive material
Cost considerations	Capital building
	Capital equipment

TABLE 1. CRITERIA TO CONSIDER WHEN IMPLEMENTING NEW RADIATION TREATMENT TECHNOLOGIES [16][a] (cont.)

Criteria	Considerations
	Personnel/operation
	Quality control equipment
	Immobilization devices
	Consumables (e.g. immobilization devices)
	Maintenance/service (of machine, ancillary machine equipment, other devices, including some quality control equipment)
	Recurring calibration of dosimetric systems
	Possible replacement of devices (e.g. dosimetric and safety equipment)
Staffing levels	Number and competence of radiation therapists
	Number and competence of medical physicists
	Number and competence of radiation oncologists

[a] Adapted from Ref. [16] with permission.
[b] IMRT: intensity modulated radiotherapy.
[c] VMAT: volumetric arc therapy.
[d] IGRT: image guided radiotherapy.

If intensity modulated radiotherapy (IMRT) and image guided radiotherapy (IGRT) are used routinely, the need for electron beams decreases for some cases (e.g. head and neck cancers). It should be noted that beam energies above 10 MV have the potential for generating a low level of neutrons, which needs to be considered from a radiation protection perspective. For some skin cancer treatments, orthovoltage X rays are an effective alternative option, providing good cosmesis.

From a physics perspective, the dose from megavoltage beams builds up to reach a maximum dose at a depth that is dependent on the beam energy; the higher the energy, the deeper the buildup depth (see Fig. 2) [35]. Sometimes a deeper buildup depth helps spare superficial normal tissues; sometimes it reduces dose uniformity in the target volume, depending on the location of the tissues at risk, such as demonstrated by Fortin et al. [26] for a head and neck study. Buildup depth is also dependent on the obliquity of beam incidence. For example, the buildup depth is reduced for oblique incidence used for breast treatment and results in a higher skin dose than if the beam is directed normally to the skin surface.

With higher energies, parallel-opposed beams provide uniform dose distributions to centrally located target volumes, especially for larger patient thicknesses (>20 cm). For smaller patient thicknesses (≤20 cm), the higher energy gain is marginal. However, using more beams with lower energies will mitigate the amount of dose variation. For instance, with IMRT or rotational techniques, there is little to be gained from using energies higher than 6 MV since the beams are generally entering the patient from multiple directions. In fact, moving to even higher beam energies (i.e. above 10 MV) could be a disadvantage due to reduced beam modulation, increased collimator transmission and neutron contamination [36]. Based on these observations, the International Commission on Radiation Units and Measurements has stated that the use of higher energy beams is not justified for IMRT [37].

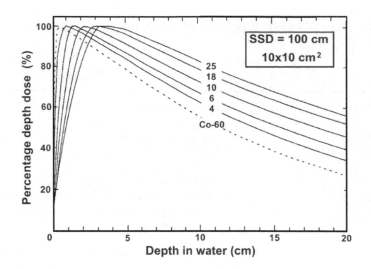

FIG. 2. Percentage depth dose curves in water for a 10 cm × 10 cm field at a source to surface distance of 100 cm for various megavoltage photon beams ranging from ^{60}Co γ rays to 25 MV X rays (reproduced from Ref. [35]).

5.2. RADIATION BEAM PROFILE CHARACTERISTICS

The distance over which the dose falls off rapidly at the edge of the radiation beam is referred to as the beam penumbra. Beam penumbras tend to be smaller for linacs than for ^{60}Co when considered in water-like tissues. However, in lungs and other regions of low density, the penumbra increases with increasing energy.

When photons interact, they generate scattered photons and electrons. Conventional linac beams have built-in flattening filters in the head of the machine to generate a uniform beam at a given depth. Due to the lack of flattening filters and more oblique scatter, ^{60}Co beams tend to have more rounded dose profiles than linacs, which is especially noticeable for larger field sizes. This can be mitigated, if necessary, using good treatment planning techniques. The same principle can be applied to some modern linac beams, which are not equipped with a flattening filter and are known as flattening filter free (FFF) beams.

5.3. TREATMENT PLAN CONSIDERATIONS

Few dose distribution comparisons between ^{60}Co and linacs have been formally published, despite widespread application. Adams and Warrington [38] compared a range of conformal and intensity modulated techniques and found that it is possible to plan high quality radiotherapy treatment for ^{60}Co, although an equivalent well designed beam blocking/compensation system or multileaf collimator (MLC) would be required, as for the linac treatment. To generate shaped fields, shielding techniques with lead blocks or a low melting point alloy can be used on both ^{60}Co machines and linacs. One general guideline is that the more beams that are used per treatment plan, the less noticeable the effect of different energies [16, 39].

5.4. MACHINE CHARACTERISTICS

The ^{60}Co dose rate is dependent on source activity and reduces at the rate of about 1% per month, or more precisely, 50% over 5.27 years. This requires a regular adjustment of the machine treatment times to maintain accurate dose delivery. A 370 TBq (10 kCi) source (a common source activity purchased with the machine or delivered on source replacement) generates outputs of approximately 2.6 Gy/min at 80 cm or 1.7 Gy/min at 100 cm. In the IAEA publication dealing with the setting up of a radiotherapy programme [15], it is advised that the minimum reference dose rate for a ^{60}Co beam is not allowed to fall below 0.4 Gy/min for a 10 cm × 10 cm field at the depth of dose maximum with the phantom surface at the isocentre. Linacs usually operate at a constant dose rate of between 2 and 6 Gy/min, sometimes with a high dose rate mode that can be greater than 20 Gy/min. A low dose rate mode is offered by some manufacturers that is typically around 0.5 Gy/min and is used for whole body radiation.

The source to collimator distance is a relevant parameter for patient set-ups. A longer source to collimator distance reduces the space between the collimator and the isocentre, and may limit patient set-ups, especially for large patients. A shorter distance between collimator and isocentre may also impede machine rotation if bulky immobilization devices such as breast boards are used.

The isocentre height from the floor determines the height to which patients are normally set up. The higher the height, the more difficult it is for shorter radiation therapists (RTTs) to see the reference marks and the light field on the patient. Typical isocentre heights range between 1.16 m for 80 cm source to axis distance (SAD) ^{60}Co machines and 1.36 m for 100 cm SAD ^{60}Co machines, with C-arm linac isocentre heights lying somewhere in-between, usually 1.24–1.30 m. Awareness of isocentre heights and patient set-up issues may impact choices made about the technology that is to be purchased.

5.5. RADIOTHERAPY TECHNIQUE OPTIONS

The following techniques and capabilities are options available for purchase on standard single energy linacs, complex multienergy linacs and some models of ^{60}Co machines [40, 41]: MLCs for beam shaping, IMRT capable, IGRT capable and volumetric arc therapy (VMAT) capable. In addition, complex multienergy linacs have options for a high dose rate mode and FFF beams. Other more advanced techniques are available for complex multienergy linacs and multisource ^{60}Co machines, including beam gating to account for the breathing motion of the patient, stereotactic radio surgery for brain tumours and stereotactic body radiotherapy, mainly for lung or liver tumours.

Additional IT infrastructure needs to be provided for all modern equipment, especially if MLC based IMRT and/or IGRT [42] are to be implemented.

6. INFRASTRUCTURE

One of the first questions that needs to be addressed when determining whether to purchase linacs or ^{60}Co machines is whether the appropriate physical infrastructure is in place to support the continued use of the treatment technology over its 10–15 year lifetime.

Infrastructure requirements for ^{60}Co machines and linacs have been described in various publications [12, 15]. Cobalt-60 machines require minimal infrastructure with standard electrical requirements. The units can be operated using an uninterruptable power supply for up to 30 minutes or battery backup for 4–6 hours. They may require air-conditioning, depending on humidity and ambient temperature. The requirements for linacs are more extensive, including three-phase mains power for the klystron or magnetron power supply, power conditioning (e.g. ±10%), voltage regulators to maintain stable voltage (e.g. ≤7%), chilled water for system cooling and an air compressor to drive the target. Also, 24 hour air-conditioning is required to maintain equipment at a constant temperature to ensure constant output, reduce humidity and remove ozone created during operation [12]. Generally, ^{60}Co machines are more robust and easier to maintain in an environment that is challenged in terms of regular and stable power, reliability of air-conditioning and water supply, and a dusty or damp atmosphere.

6.1. TREATMENT ROOM DESIGN

6.1.1. Shielding

Shielding considerations are dependent on the highest beam energy, the maximum dose rate, the amount of time the beam is on, the beam directions when in use and the occupancy of adjacent areas. Using a ^{60}Co machine bunker to accommodate a linac will generally require significant shielding alterations as higher energies require more shielding. In addition, there may be differences in the footprint of the machine. For typical concrete wall thicknesses of density 2.35 g/cm^3, primary beam barriers can range between 1.38 m and 2.32 m for ^{60}Co and 10 MV X rays, respectively, with secondary scatter barriers being approximately half those values [15]. Linacs with energies above 10 MV require specialized neutron shielding, generally using borated materials to decelerate and capture neutrons.

If new bunkers are built, a generic design is recommended that is based on the highest likely future requirements in terms of maximum photon energy (e.g. up to 10 MV) and workload [22]. Whether alterations are made to an existing bunker or a new bunker is built, full shielding calculations need to be performed by a medical physicist and are dependent on the local circumstances. Hence, a medical physicist needs to be involved in the facility planning process well before a cancer treatment centre is constructed. From a structural engineering perspective, quality control of the poured concrete is required at the time of construction, to ensure that uniform concrete density is achieved.

6.1.2. Maze and entry door

A longer maze can reduce the shielding and thickness of the entrance door or entirely exclude the need for it to be shielded. However, longer mazes increase the overall footprint of the bunker and could add to the volume of concrete required. Again, it is likely that higher energies will require more concrete. Generally, the smaller the maze, the more shielding will be required in the door. Heavy shielded doors bring their own substantial costs, as well as concerns about short term and long term maintenance. Furthermore, heavy doors add to the patient's overall booking time, since these doors generally open and close relatively slowly. This slow responsiveness also has the disadvantage of being a hindrance in the event of a medical emergency. It is important to have a backup system to open the shielded door to allow access in case of the failure or loss of electrical power. For these reasons, a larger maze is preferred, reducing or removing the need for doors to be used for shielding purposes, depending on the room design [22, 43]. It is important to note that both the door and the maze need to be wide enough to deliver equipment and patients on stretchers.

6.1.3. Room dimensions

Necessary room dimensions are dependent on the specific technologies purchased. Linacs require additional space for electronics cabinets and modulators, and thus usually require more space than ^{60}Co machines. The fully extended couch rotation needs to be accommodated for all C-arm radiotherapy machines, a fact that is sometimes overlooked by architects with no experience in designing radiation treatment rooms. In addition, storage space in the treatment room for set-up aids, devices and accessories is also essential. The use of special techniques at extended distances, such as large field treatments, is another consideration. Floor thicknesses need to be addressed, especially if a pit is required for the base frame of the machine. If new bunkers are built, they could be designed for a 100 cm SAD high energy machine to ensure the future accommodation of such a machine, even if it is not in the present plan. The most generic design for a radiotherapy department can be found in Ref. [22].

In 1995, Glasgow and Corrigan [44] compared the cost of upgrading an existing bunker with an 80 cm SAD ^{60}Co machine to house a 6 MV C-arm machine or a 100 cm SAD ^{60}Co machine, and found that the upgrade for the higher energy linac would cost about 37% more as a result of the additional electrical services, water cooling, air-conditioning and shielding requirements. While these general principles have not changed much, some newer linac technologies have a smaller footprint and built-in beam 'stoppers', which may result in lower primary shielding requirements.

6.1.4. Air-conditioning requirements

High energy linacs with high dose rate modes create ozone, so 2–10 air exchanges of room volume per hour are needed [22]. Air-conditioning ducts can be large and are constructed in such a way as to not compromise the shielding (such ducts might be positioned above the door and ceiling). Special shielding calculations are needed for any room ducting that potentially reduces the shielding effectiveness of the walls to ensure adequate shielding from both photons and neutrons.

6.2. MACHINE SERVICING

The purchase of both ^{60}Co machines and linacs needs to include service contracts with the manufacturer for the lifetime of the machine, with a guaranteed clinical uptime (e.g. 97% for 40 hours per week) and acceptable service response time. Local service agents are ideally readily available. Lack of such readily available servicing is a major obstacle to the successful introduction of radiotherapy [45]. Therefore, a key consideration is whether the manufacturer has appropriate machine servicing capabilities, whether servicing is affordable and whether it is easy to access. A lack of appropriate servicing could result in significant downtime [45, 46]. Typical costs for annual service contracts range between 8% and 15% of the initial total cost of the machine. Replacement parts may also be expensive, especially in some countries [45]. In LMICs, downtime is often exacerbated by a lack of local accredited maintenance expertise and import or visa delays for spare parts [45] or international service representatives.

The service is conducted by an engineer who has been trained by the machine manufacturer. However, it is also useful to have personnel in the radiotherapy department who are trained by the manufacturer to perform the first line of servicing. This allows simple problems to be resolved quickly without waiting for the manufacturer's service engineer to arrive on-site. A full tool kit on-site is therefore necessary, as well as spare parts for elements of the machine that are prone to failure. One report noted that such frontline servicing in African countries is often performed by medical physicists [45]. However, this approach is strongly discouraged, since it conflicts with the responsibility of the medical physicist to authorize the clinical use of a unit after repair.

Given the increased complexity of the linac, the maintenance required for a linac is more extensive than for a ^{60}Co machine. For example, depending on usage and number of treatment hours per day, a linac can require eight full days per year of preventative maintenance, while in an ideal environment a ^{60}Co machine requires three days per year. Catastrophic machine failures may also require recommissioning of the system [12]. Modern standard single energy linacs are more stable and can be recommissioned more rapidly. Cobalt-60, being a radioactive source, provides consistent output data, so less time is required for recommissioning following machine servicing and repair, including after a source exchange.

6.3. RADIATION SAFETY

The use of any high energy radiotherapy machine necessitates careful consideration of the safety of the patient, the staff and the public, which includes the need for physical security of any radioactive sources used in radiotherapy. Therefore, safety is ideally at the forefront of any decision on purchasing equipment. Radiotherapy needs to be provided in an environment where there is a properly established governmental, legal and regulatory framework for safety.

Safety issues have been described in detail in several IAEA publications, including Ref. [15] and in IAEA Safety Standards Series No. GSR Part 3, Radiation Protection and Safety of Radiation Sources [47].

Review of these publications indicates that compromised safety considerations have led to patient and worker harm [15, 47]. It is imperative that the facility design and structure are adequate for all types of radiotherapy equipment. This includes having shielding calculations performed by medical physicists and reviewed and confirmed by the regulatory authority prior to construction of the facility.

An appropriate number of trained and qualified staff usually undergo manufacturer specific applications training on the equipment at the facility. This training is ideally provided to all staff, but is usually provided to a core group and then disseminated internally. Misunderstanding of the use and capabilities of radiotherapy equipment has led to medical errors that have harmed patients, as described in IAEA Safety Standards Series No. SSG-46, Radiation Protection and Safety in Medical Uses of Ionizing Radiation [48]. Full mechanical use of the equipment needs to be possible without risk of collision with the patient or other equipment.

The equipment needs to be serviced regularly. Safety systems in the treatment room should always be operational and tested regularly. Under no circumstances should radiotherapy be provided in an unsafe facility where emergency switches or video and oral communications equipment are not operational. The facility needs to maintain up to date policies and procedures on how therapy is delivered, and management ideally supports a strong safety culture. This can be accomplished by having an overall management policy that supports a culture of safety, to include stopping activities that are not understood or perceived to cause harm to the worker or the patient [48]. Many of the major radiotherapy accidents that have been reported were the result of poor communication, lack of training and education, lack of policies and procedures, lack of management support for a strong safety culture or a combination of one or more of these deficiencies [49, 50].

A specific safety consideration for equipment containing radioactive sources, including ^{60}Co teletherapy, is the risk of the source remaining in the unshielded position following a treatment rather than retracting into the shielded position [47]. If this happens, safety procedures should be followed to minimize the radiation dose to the patient and staff, and staff will need to manually retract the source into the shielded position. This requires special equipment and dose monitoring capabilities. Staff need to ensure that the 'T-bar' to force the source into the shielded position is always readily available. Emergency response training for staff is ideally repeated annually. If the emergency procedures are activated, occupational exposure should be reviewed immediately and patient dose estimations performed. The machine needs to be serviced before continued use.

6.4. STAFFING CONSIDERATIONS

Staffing levels in a radiotherapy facility are dependent on the quantity and complexity of equipment, the number of patients, the types of procedures, and education and training requirements. The IAEA has produced a quantitative algorithm that determines recommended staffing levels based on all these factors [51]. This demonstrates that fewer staff are required when mainly conventional two dimensional (2-D) techniques, with a small percentage of 3-D conformal radiotherapy (3-D CRT), are used on a single energy megavoltage beam unit, be it ^{60}Co or a linac. However, the addition of advanced technologies does not necessarily result in a pro rata increase in staffing. In terms of the competence level required for 2-D treatments versus, for example, IMRT, more detailed knowledge of the technology and procedures is required. However, simpler technologies have their own challenges; it is therefore difficult to imply that a lower level of competence is required for simpler technologies. Detailed knowledge and skills in more complex technologies may not be required when only conventional techniques are practised. A component of 3-D CRT is always highly desirable. Previous IAEA reports give clear descriptions of the additional knowledge required as the range of cancer types being treated with more sophisticated techniques expands [42, 52].

7. EQUIPMENT OTHER
THAN TREATMENT MACHINES

This publication discusses the considerations necessary when selecting a megavoltage treatment machine. However, as indicated in Appendix I, the process of radiotherapy is complex and involves multiple steps and multiple technologies. It is not possible to offer radiotherapy by procuring an external beam radiotherapy treatment machine only, as other equipment is needed. Appendix III gives details of a standard equipment package for a radiotherapy department. This section summarizes which equipment other than the treatment machine is included in such a package.

7.1. PRETREATMENT IMAGING

To irradiate malignant tissues while minimizing the dose to healthy structures, the precise location of the malignant tissues and the critical normal tissue structures needs to be known. In 2-D radiotherapy this is often handled with a conventional simulator. However, for more precise tumour and normal tissue localization using 3-D CRT, a CT scanner will be needed [52]. The CT scanner could be housed in the diagnostic imaging department and used part of the time for radiation treatment planning. If used for treatment planning, the CT scanner needs to have a flat-top couch, slice and positioning indicators, and a direct connection to the treatment planning system. While this is the least expensive approach for CT imaging, a dedicated CT simulator could be considered for therapy planning purposes in the radiotherapy department should there be a significant number of 3-D cases. Some method of imaging the patient is an essential part of the armamentarium of the entire radiation treatment process. Other useful imaging methods for treatment planning are magnetic resonance imaging and positron emission tomography imaging, although the need for their availability is dependent on the main types of cancer being treated, local financial resources, and access to other imaging and nuclear medicine departments.

7.2. RADIATION TREATMENT PLANNING SYSTEM

Like imaging for radiotherapy, a computerized radiation treatment planning system (TPS) is an essential technology [52]. If the department is expanding techniques to include IMRT, the existing TPS may have to be upgraded with one that is appropriate for the required planning technique [42]. The medical physicist is responsible for establishing the technical aspects involved in the TPS upgrade, including its acceptance testing and commissioning [15], whereas the head of the clinic or of the department is usually responsible for finding the funds to pay for the upgrade.

7.3. ONCOLOGY INFORMATION SYSTEM

For imaging, beam shaping and beam modifying devices, a dedicated departmental IT infrastructure is needed for transmitting and storing the data from the treatment planning and delivery systems. For example, if an MLC is installed, the MLC leaf configurations as determined on the TPS have to be transmitted from the TPS to the delivery system for reasons of safety and efficiency. For this, a record and verify system (RVS) is needed as part of the departmental oncology information system [53].

For clinical, administrative and possible scientific issues, it is important that there is a provision for adequate, well-maintained long term image and data archiving linked to these systems, and a significant IT infrastructure may be required to achieve this.

7.4. UNINTERRUPTABLE POWER SUPPLY

The availability of an uninterruptable power supply is essential for IT systems and linacs, as some environments are prone to power fluctuations.

7.5. ANCILLARY EQUIPMENT

Associated ancillary equipment must also be considered when purchasing new major equipment or introducing new radiotherapy techniques. Examples include (a) 3-D dosimetry phantoms needed for acceptance testing, commissioning and quality control (QC) of treatment machines [15]; (b) radiation detectors such as ionization chambers, diodes, in vivo dosimeters and radiation protection survey meters; (c) QC devices for general machine quality assurance (QA) of the radiation treatment technologies, as well as equipment for patient-specific dosimetry; and (d) devices and consumables associated with patient immobilization.

8. COST CONSIDERATIONS

8.1. COST ESTIMATION

When planning a new or expanded department, not only the upfront costs of developing a new facility have to be addressed, including the costs of construction, equipment and the training of new staff, but also the operating costs of delivering treatments for the lifetime of the machines once the facility is established [1, 12, 54]. The estimation of costs for a new department or an expansion is dependent on local circumstances. When procuring a machine, the lifetime cost of the machine needs to be considered. If funds are not available to cover the lifetime costs, which include the initial purchase of the machine, annual maintenance, consumables, staff, etc., a cheaper machine is advisable.

The relative component costs (of the building, equipment and personnel) very much depend on a country's income level [1]. These costs vary dramatically by region in the world, although capital equipment costs have the smallest regional variation. Relative component costs show that equipment is the major relative cost in low income countries (81%) while salaries are the major relative cost in high income countries (64%). Costs are impacted by factors such as facility size, level of treatment complexity, construction costs, staff costs, and clinical operating conditions such as the length of the working day and the time allocated for different activities.

The IAEA has produced several reports and calculators that can aid in such cost calculations [51, 55]. A number of considerations need to be taken into account when estimating the lifetime cost of a new machine in a radiotherapy department.

These consist of the following:

(a)   Capital costs associated with the land and construction;
(b)   Capital costs associated with the purchase of the treatment and imaging machines;
(c)   Service contracts with the manufacturers for all machines in the department;
(d)   Dosimetry and QC equipment (including maintenance and calibration);
(e)   Immobilization devices (including their replacement);
(f)   Additional ancillary equipment;
(g)   Consumable items;
(h)   Operating costs;
(i)   Building maintenance costs;

(j)   Taxes;

(k)   Staff salaries;

(l)   Continuous education and training of staff;

(m) Research, if any;

(n)   Decommissioning costs at the end of the machine's lifetime, especially for ^{60}Co sources.

One way of saving costs for ^{60}Co teletherapy machines is to have both 100 cm SAD and 80 cm SAD units. A higher activity source from the 100 cm SAD unit can be cascaded to the shorter SAD machine after a period of decay, thereby reducing the total cost of source exchanges. Therefore, only one source needs to be procured for the two machines every five years, which results in a significant cost saving over the lifetime of the machines.

Healy et al. [12] performed a relative cost analysis in 2016, looking specifically at machine capital and maintenance costs over a 15 year period of operation, but did not include building capital costs or personnel operating costs. The results are shown in Table 2 and have been updated. These estimates are dependent on the vendor of a specific machine, but it is expected that the relative costs of the different machines given in Table 2 will be similar in each country. Such relative cost estimates are performed by the strategic task force prior to the actual purchase.

While the data shown in Table 2 address machine related procurement and maintenance costs, they do not address any of the other components associated with the operation of a radiotherapy programme. The time-driven, activity based cost analysis of Van Dyk et al. [54] gives a very detailed description of all the cost factors associated with a radiotherapy department, from capital costs related to constructing the entire facility to staffing costs and equipment operating costs. Furthermore, it demonstrates that the equipment associated with a radiotherapy programme includes much more than the external beam radiotherapy machines that are summarized in Table 2. Tables 3–5 indicate the costs associated with human resources (Table 3), the costs associated with equipment (Table 4) and the costs associated with building (Table 5). Note that the numbers are representative of the data used in their analysis and give an indication of factors to consider. The currency used in Table 2 is different from that used in Tables 3–5, since the data in the tables are drawn from different publications. To obtain an overall cost estimate, the appropriate currency conversion will be needed. Furthermore, since salaries vary significantly among high income, upper middle income, lower middle income and low income countries, in Table 3 only the extremes of the cost factors associated with human resources in high income and low income countries are provided. For planning purposes, quotations should be obtained for local circumstances.

Tables 3–5 refer to countries with different per capita economic income levels, such as high income, low income and LMIC, but income levels can vary substantially even within individual countries, as pointed out by Zubizarreta et al. [56]. Thus, estimations performed will need to consider the local income parameters.

8.2. CALCULATION OF THE REQUIRED NUMBER OF TREATMENT MACHINES

Before the number and types of treatment machines can be determined, basic information is needed on the number and types of patients with specific disease diagnoses, the disease stages, the number of patients requiring curative treatment and the number requiring palliative treatment. This information can be found in the national cancer registry, or, if one does not exist, from data given in GLOBOCAN [21]. The next stage is to develop draft clinical protocols that define the types of radiotherapy techniques needed and the numbers of treatment fractions required for each specific technique. These broad protocols will help in deciding which machine is to be purchased. Once the technology is in place, the protocols need to be developed in more detail, including clear instructions for all the steps in the process, from pretreatment imaging to treatment delivery. A detailed template for protocol development has been described by Nilsson et al. [57].

TABLE 2. COSTS OF PURCHASING AND MAINTAINING Co-60 MACHINES AND LINACS OVER A 15 YEAR PERIOD [12][a]

Cost category	Costs (€)		
	Co-60 machine with RVS[b], excluding MLC[c] and EPID[d]	6 MV linac with MLC, EPID and RVS (excluding IMRT[e])	Complex multienergy linac (including electrons) with MLC, EPID and RVS (excluding IMRT)
Upfront cost, including one year of warranty	600 000	900 000	1 500 000
14 year service contract	500 000	1 260 000	2 100 000
Source exchanges (two)	500 000	n.a.[f]	n.a.
Total cost over 15 years	1 600 000	2 160 000	3 600 000

[a] Adapted from Ref. [12] with permission.
[b] RVS: record and verify system.
[c] MLC: multileaf collimator.
[d] EPID: electronic portal imaging device.
[e] IMRT: intensity modulated radiotherapy.
[f] n.a.: not applicable.

TABLE 3. COST FACTORS ASSOCIATED WITH HUMAN RESOURCES AND TYPICAL TIME SPENT BY PERSONNEL ON NON-CLINICAL DUTIES [54][a, b]

Role	Costs (US $)[c]				Typical time spent on non-clinical duties (%)
	Training cost per person		Monthly salary per FTE[d]		
	High income country	Low income country	High income country	Low income country	
Radiation oncologist	550 000	100 000	17 000	696	40
Medical physicist	225 000	50 000	9 165	375	20
Radiation therapist	66 858	28 000	4 842	197	5
Nurse	66 858	28 000	4 603	256	5
Engineer	150 000	33 333	6 110	250	5

[a] Selected data from table 1 of Ref. [54].
[b] This assumes a working day of 8 hours with 28 days of annual leave.
[c] Only the extremes of high income and low income countries are provided.
[d] FTE: full time equivalent.

TABLE 4. CAPITAL RESOURCE COSTS RELATED TO RADIOTHERAPY EQUIPMENT FOR HIGH INCOME COUNTRIES AND LOW AND MIDDLE INCOME COUNTRIES [54][a]

Equipment	Purchase price (US $)	Operational parameters[b]	
		Lifetime (years)	Annual amortization (%)
Additional CBCT[c] to the linac	350 000	12	8.3
CT[d] simulator	409 000	12	8.3
Treatment planning system	272 000	5	20
Record and verify/oncology management system	130 000	5	20
High dose rate afterloader	545 000	12	8.3
3-D brachytherapy treatment planning system	Included in afterloader price	5	20

[a] Selected data from table 1 of Ref. [54].
[b] It is assumed that 10% of the operational time is dedicated to maintenance and that all equipment is available for operation for 12 hours per day.
[c] CBCT: cone-beam computed tomography.
[d] CT: computed tomography.

TABLE 5. CONSTRUCTION COSTS RELATED TO RADIOTHERAPY EQUIPMENT [54][a]

Facility	Purchase price (US $)[b]	
	High income country	Low and middle income country
Reception + other administrative/public areas (10% of total) (250 m^2 + 122 m^2)	1 027 666	459 600
Consultation area (277 m^2)	743 246	332 400
Treatment preparation (simulation, planning) (332 m^2)	890 858	398 400
Linac bunker (141 m^2)	567 497	253 800
Brachytherapy area (189 m^2)	608 550	272 160

[a] Selected data from table 1 of Ref. [54].
[b] Based on 2% annual maintenance cost and 3.33% annual amortization, assuming a 30 year lifetime and 12 hour working day.

Once an estimate of the number of treatment fractions to be delivered by radiotherapy per year and the broad treatment protocols have been established, the next step is to determine the levels of complexity of the treatment techniques that will be used, since this will determine the overall time per fraction, which in turn will determine the number of machines required. While 2-D techniques may be adequate for most palliative and some radical treatments, and are generally the fastest and most efficient to deliver, Ref. [1] defines three levels of complexity for the more advanced treatment techniques, each requiring that the patient is in the treatment room for a different length of time per fraction: (a) 3-D CRT at 15 mins per fraction, (b) 3-D CRT with IGRT at 18 mins per fraction, and (c) IMRT with IGRT at 24 mins per fraction. Note that the actual irradiation time is only one component of the patient's total time in the treatment room and the times quoted above refer to the time the patient enters and leaves the treatment room, including set-up time, imaging time (if applicable), irradiation time and patient exit time. Clearly, there will be individual variations depending on the nature and location of the disease, the prescription and patient specific circumstances (e.g. mobility, level of pain, need for sedation).

The disease types and numbers are needed to determine the average number of treatment fractions, which determine the workload and the required number of treatment machines. This recognizes that curative patients for different diseases may require different numbers of fractions and that radical courses generally require more fractions than palliative courses. A number of publications and databases provide guidance on determining radiotherapy needs [15, 17, 21]. Appendices IV and V give a detailed description of how to determine the number of treatment machines that are required in a department based on the known number of patients to be treated and further input data, including average numbers of fractions per treatment course and the average in-room patient time required for each treatment.

The parameters required for performing the calculation for the determination of numbers of machines include the following:

(a)   Total number of patients to be treated per year;
(b)   Average number of treatment fractions per patient;
(c)   Total number of treatment fractions per year;
(d)   Number of operational hours per day;
(e)   Number of treatment days per year;
(f)   Number of treatment fractions per hour.

9. SUMMARY OF THE COMPARISON BETWEEN ^{60}Co MACHINES AND LINACS

Table 6 summarizes various aspects to consider that relate to the choice of ^{60}Co machines, standard single energy linacs and complex multienergy linacs. It is advisable that departments with more than one machine could have one or more single energy units, be they ^{60}Co machines or low energy linacs (e.g. 4 or 6 MV) for 2-D and 3-D CRT, and more sophisticated linacs with IMRT and IGRT capabilities for more advanced treatments [58]. For larger departments with more than one machine, machine (beam energy) matching could be considered such that if one machine fails, another machine can absorb the workload of that machine.

TABLE 6. SUMMARY OF FACTORS COMPARING Co-60 MACHINES AND LINACS

Issue	Co-60 machine	Standard single energy linac	Complex multienergy linac	Comments
Clinical considerations				
Technique capability	2-D and 3-D CRT[a]	2-D radiotherapy, 3-D CRT, IMRT[b]	More advanced techniques possible such as IMRT, VMAT[c] and IGRT[d]	— Complexity dependent on disease types and staging, availability of resources and properly trained staff
Radiation beam characteristics				
Penumbra	>1 cm	~1 cm	~1 cm	— Dependent on source diameter — Dependent on linac energy and technique — Dependent on tissue density — Significance depends on uncertainty in target volume definition — Significance depends on patient set-up uncertainty — Significance depends on organ motion — Biological penumbra is always sharper than physical penumbra (i.e. reducing the significance of a larger physical penumbra)
Beam penetration (PDD[f] at 10 cm depth)	56.4% (80 cm SSD[e]) 58.7% (100 cm SSD)	67.5% (6 MV) 63.0% (4 MV)	67.5% (6 MV) 73.0% (10 MV) 79.0% (18 MV)	— Lower energy is better for target volumes near skin surface (e.g. head and neck) — Lower energies are useful for smaller patients (e.g. paediatric). Impact of lower energy can be reduced by use of multifield techniques
Scattering/dose uniformity	Less flat beams at depth	Flattening filtered beams	Flattening filtered beams Optional: FFF[g] beam	— Minor effect for small fields — Can be reduced by use of flattening filters, compensators and more complex treatment planning for larger fields — Increased out of field dose when IMRT techniques with larger numbers of monitor units are used — Additional shielding considerations when using higher dose rates and larger number of monitor units

TABLE 6. SUMMARY OF FACTORS COMPARING Co-60 MACHINES AND LINACS (cont.)

Issue	Co-60 machine	Standard single energy linac	Complex multienergy linac	Comments
Depth of maximum dose (d_{max})	0.5 cm	1.5 cm (6 MV) 1.0 cm (4 MV)	1.5 cm (6 MV) 2.5 cm (10 MV) 3.5 cm (18 MV)	— Dependent on field size and SSD — Larger fields and shorter SSDs give shorter d_{max} and higher skin doses
Dose variations due to contours and tissue inhomogeneities	Significant	Lower with increasing energies	Lower with increasing energies	— Lack of electronic equilibrium in high energy photon beams in lung yields larger penumbral effects — Tissue/bone or tissue/prosthesis interface effects extend over a larger volume in higher energy photon beams due to longer electron ranges
Relative dose to bone	0.96 (small beams) 1.14 (large beams)	0.97 (6 MV, small beams) 1.10 (6 MV, large beams)	0.97 (6 MV, small beams) 1.10 (6 MV, large beams) 1.00 (18 MV, small beams) 1.04 (18 MV, large beams)	— Difference is relatively small for conventional field sizes when considering photon spectrum at depth for a range of energies — Large field Co-60 has potential advantage for TBI[h] for bone marrow transplants and large field techniques for treatment of bone metastases
Machine characteristics				
Dose rate	~2.60 Gy/min with new source ~1.25 Gy/min after 5 years	1.00–6.00 Gy/min	2.00–6.00 Gy/min Up to 25 Gy/min in high dose rate mode	— Co-60 has lower uncertainty in dose delivery since it is not dependent on a monitor ion chamber or a beam steering system — Co-60 dose rates are dependent on initial source activity and could be as high as 2.6 Gy/min
Patient collimator distance	~30 cm for 80 cm SAD ~50 cm for 100 cm SAD	~50 cm	~50 cm	— Larger distance better for patient set-up — Larger distance increases penumbra — Practically, a compromise between large and small distance
Isocentre height above the floor	~115 cm ~130–136 cm (100 SAD)	124–134 cm	124–134 cm	— Traditionally smaller on Co-60 machines — Low isocentre advantageous for shorter radiation therapists

TABLE 6. SUMMARY OF FACTORS COMPARING Co-60 MACHINES AND LINACS (cont.)

Issue	Co-60 machine	Standard single energy linac	Complex multienergy linac	Comments
Photon source	— Radioactive decay — Dose rate reduces by ~1% per month or 50% over 5.27 years	— X rays from target — Constant dose rate	— X rays from target — Constant dose rate	— Co-60 requires source change every 5–7 years — More monoenergetic for Co-60 — simplifies dose calibrations and calculations — Co-60 has reduced beam hardening in attenuators
Options				
Beam shaping/MLCs[j]	Not standard	Optional	Standard	— Blocks on shielding trays can be used on both Co-60 machines and linacs — MLCs are routinely available on most linacs and are optional on some Co-60 machines
IMRT capable	Not standard	Optional	Optional	
VMAT capable	Not standard	Not standard	Optional	
IGRT capable	Not standard	Optional (MV imaging)	Optional (MV and kV imaging)	
High dose rate mode/ FFF machines	High dose rate mode not available	Not standard	Optional	— FFF option on linacs give higher dose rate
Record and verify system/oncology information system	Optional	Optional	Standard	— Necessary when an MLC is used to shape the field
Infrastructure/service/maintenance issues				
Local infrastructure	Single phase, simple power source	Three phase, stable power source	Three phase, stable power source	— Linacs have more stringent requirements — Linacs may require power conditioner

TABLE 6. SUMMARY OF FACTORS COMPARING Co-60 MACHINES AND LINACS (cont.)

Issue	Co-60 machine	Standard single energy linac	Complex multienergy linac	Comments
Room requirements	Simple	May require air-conditioning and chilled water	Require air-conditioning and chilled water	— Review special techniques such as TBI, since this may require a larger room
Shielding	Lower energy, therefore less thick walls required	Wall thicknesses dependent on maximum beam energy	Wall thicknesses dependent on maximum beam energy	— Linacs greater than 10 MeV have increased personnel exposures due to residual activity and neutron production — Linacs greater than 10 MeV have increased patient dose equivalent due to neutron production — Co-60 has head leakage with beam off of less than 0.2%
Service availability/ issues	Essential	Essential	Essential	— Important to have both service personnel and parts readily available for either Co-60 or linacs — Downtime is similar now for Co-60 and standard single energy linacs with no EPID[j] or MLC — Options such as MLC, IMRT, IGRT increase downtime
IT infrastructure	Basic	Important	Important	— An oncology information management system is critical for transfer of image and treatment planning data, as well as patient records
Safety/security considerations				
Transport/disposal issues	Source transport issues Source disposal issues	No concern	Minor concern	— The Co-60 concerns can be handled with appropriate organization and training — The long term activation of some parts of a complex multienergy linac head needs adequate managing during decommissioning
Emergency situations related to source retraction	Stuck source issues	n.a.[k]	n.a.	— The Co-60 concerns can be handled through unique safety considerations including specialized equipment and occupational exposure monitoring equipment

TABLE 6. SUMMARY OF FACTORS COMPARING Co-60 MACHINES AND LINACS (cont.)

Issue	Co-60 machine	Standard single energy linac	Complex multienergy linac	Comments
Ozone	Minor risk	Minor risk with adequate air-conditioning	Higher risk especially with electron beams and high dose rates	
Cost considerations				
Capital building	Lower than linac	Dependent on maximum beam energy	Dependent on maximum beam energy	— Consider designing Co-60 room for possible linac use for future replacement
Capital equipment	Co-60 somewhat less expensive	Cost dependent on maximum linac energy and the added options such as MLC, IMRT, IGRT	Cost dependent on maximum linac energy and the added options such as MLC, IMRT, VMAT, IGRT, kV imaging, MV imaging	— Need to consider additional equipment for both Co-60 and linac — Simulator — Treatment planning system — Dosimetry/QA devices — Phantoms — Radiation protection tools
Personnel/operating	Somewhat less staffing if simpler techniques are used	Staffing levels dependent on technology and technique complexity	Staffing levels dependent on technology and technique complexity	— Radiation oncologists: depends on number of patients — Medical physicists: depends on number of patients, number of machines and complexity of techniques — Radiation therapists: depends on number of treatment hours per day — IT personnel for computer/network integration — Oncology nurses
Maintenance/service	Full service contract required	Full service contract required	Full service contract required	— In-house service/maintenance personnel for first line of servicing — Service contracts approximately 10–15% of cost of machine per year

TABLE 6. SUMMARY OF FACTORS COMPARING Co-60 MACHINES AND LINACS (cont.)

Issue	Co-60 machine	Standard single energy linac	Complex multienergy linac	Comments
Staffing considerations				
Number of staff	Fewer for less complex techniques	More for IMRT and IGRT	More for IMRT, IGRT and 4-D	— Additional training required for more sophisticated techniques

a   CRT: conformal radiotherapy.
b   IMRT: intensity modulated radiotherapy.
c   VMAT: volumetric arc therapy.
d   IGRT: image guided radiotherapy.
e   SSD: source to surface distance.
f   PDD: percentage depth dose.
g   FFF: flattening filter free.
h   TBI: total body irradiation.
i   MLC: multileaf collimator.
j   EPID: electronic portal imaging devices.
k   n.a.: not applicable.

Appendix I

STEPS IN A TYPICAL RADIATION TREATMENT PROCESS, TECHNOLOGIES USED AT EACH STAGE AND PROFESSIONAL STAFF TYPICALLY INVOLVED

The process of radiation treatment is complex and involves multiple steps, from the initial diagnosis to the post-treatment follow up of the patient. Multiple technologies and clinical protocols are involved at each one of these stages, and a number of different specialized professional staff are employed. In Table 7 an overview of the steps of the typical radiation treatment process is provided, including specifications regarding the technologies and professional staff involved.

TABLE 7. STEPS IN THE TYPICAL RADIATION TREATMENT PROCESS, TECHNOLOGIES AT EACH STAGE AND PROFESSIONAL STAFF TYPICALLY INVOLVED

Step in radiation treatment process	Technologies involved	Professional staff
Diagnosis	Pathology laboratory	Pathologist
Patient assessment for the decision to treat using radiotherapy	Diagnostic imaging technologies, pathology laboratory	Diagnostic radiologist, radiation oncologist, pathologist
Imaging for target volume and organ at risk determination	Simulator, CT[a] simulator, MRI[b], PET[c] imaging	RTT[d], diagnostic radiology technologist, medical physicist
Immobilization and positioning of the patient for treatment	Simulator, immobilization devices	RTT
Initial treatment planning directives to include dose prescription to the tumour and organs at risk, motion management protocol	Treatment protocols	Radiation oncologist
Delineation or localization of target volumes	Patient images imported into a treatment planning system	Radiation oncologist
Delineation or localization of organs at risk	Simulator, treatment planning system	Radiation oncologist, medical physicist
Development of radiation treatment plan	Computerized treatment planning system	RTT, medical physicist
Pretreatment review	Treatment planning system	Radiation oncologist, medical physicist
Plan evaluation	Treatment planning system	Radiation oncologist, medical physicist
Plan approval	Treatment planning system	Radiation oncologist
Plan verification	Dosimetry phantoms to simulate patient-specific dose delivery	Medical physicist

TABLE 7. STEPS IN THE TYPICAL RADIATION TREATMENT PROCESS, TECHNOLOGIES AT EACH STAGE AND PROFESSIONAL STAFF TYPICALLY INVOLVED (cont.)

Step in radiation treatment process	Technologies involved	Professional staff
Set-up and image review as necessary	Port films, electronic portal imaging, image guidance technologies	RTT, radiation oncologist, medical physicist
Dose delivery for each treatment fraction	kV X ray machines, Co-60 machines, linacs, brachytherapy	RTT, radiation oncologist
Post-treatment review	Diagnostic imaging	Radiation oncologist

Note: The details of this process are dependent on the specific clinical protocol and can vary by disease site, institution and the specific technologies available in the department.

[a] CT: computed tomography.

[b] MRI: magnetic resonance imaging.

[c] PET: positron emission tomography.

[d] RTT: radiation therapist.

Appendix II

QUESTIONS TO CONSIDER IN THE IMPLEMENTATION OF MEGAVOLTAGE RADIATION TREATMENT TECHNOLOGIES

The following questions are designed to assist organizations that are considering the implementation of new radiation treatment technologies or the replacement of existing technologies. For some of the questions, references are included to provide guidance in terms of addressing the answer to the question.

A. Administrative and regulatory issues

(1) Is there a radiation regulatory infrastructure in the country [47]?
(2) Is there a strategic task force in place that is managed by the national health authorities?
(3) Is there a national cancer control plan to guide implementation of the new centre(s) [17]?
(4) Has the design been approved and authorization been given to construct the facility?
(5) Have the correct licences been obtained from the regulatory authority for the operation of the facility and the equipment?

B. Equipment selection and customization

(1) Is there a core implementation team in place to address the purchase of new radiotherapy technology [15, 20, 22]?
(2) What types of cancer diagnoses are predominant [17]?
(3) What are the number of radical and palliative courses of treatment [59]?
(4) What are the number of cases and corresponding fractions that need to be treated [59, 60]?
(5) What level of complexity is likely to be used for these treatment fractions (e.g. 2-D radiotherapy, 3-D CRT, IMRT/VMAT/IGRT) [42, 52]?
(6) Is there a local/regional commitment to access the radiotherapy treatment that will be provided in the proposed centre?
(7) For limited access, is there a national prioritization strategy to select patients for radiotherapy?
(8) How many radiation treatment machines are required for the country?
(9) What are the energies and special treatment options for each of the required machines?

C. Infrastructure

(1) Has a plan been developed for the design of a new facility [15, 22]?
(2) Is a bunker available to install the machine?
(3) Are any special treatment techniques required that impact on room design or treatment machine specifications?
(4) Have the radiation shielding calculations been performed by a medical physicist?
(5) Is the appropriate infrastructure in place for ^{60}Co machines and/or linacs [12, 15]?
    (i) Is there a stable and adequate power supply for operating either ^{60}Co machines or linacs?
    (ii) Is there an appropriate chilled water supply for linacs?
    (iii) Is appropriate air-conditioning available for linacs?
    (iv) Is the infrastructure for the security of the ^{60}Co source in place [61]?
(6) Have the appropriate Radiation Safety and Radiation Quality Assurance Committees been defined with mandates and terms of reference [15, 48]?
(7) Has a plan been developed to recruit or train all the new professional staff required in the department?

(i)   Will qualified staff be available to aid with the planning and implementation process?

(8)   Are the requisite staffing levels going to be met at the time of opening the facility [15, 50]?

(9)   Have all of the required medical physicists, radiation oncologists and RTTs been trained in the new technology?

(10) Is there a safety culture in the department [50]?

D.   Equipment beyond treatment machines

(1)   What additional equipment or software is required for treatment planning (e.g. simulator, TPS, RVS, oncology information system) and is there appropriate software to allow clinical techniques to be implemented [42, 52]?

(2)   Has a list been made of all the ancillary equipment that may be required (e.g. for dosimetry, QA/QC, immobilization, in vivo dosimetry) [20]?

E.   Cost considerations

(1)   Has a full budget been developed for the lifetime of the machines?
  (i)   Have quotations been obtained from architects and builders to generate an estimate of construction and building costs?
  (ii)   Have quotations been obtained from all the vendors capable of installing the desired equipment?
  (iii)   Has an estimate been made of the operating costs?
        — Treatment machine servicing and maintenance contract;
        — Staff costs;
        — Costs of electrical power, water, heating/air-conditioning;
        — Immobilization devices;
        — QA/QC and dosimetry equipment.

(2)   Has the project gone out to tender?
  (i)   For (re)building the facilities?
  (ii)   For the purchase of the treatment technology [3]?
  (iii)   For the purchase of associated technologies for imaging and treatment planning?
  (iv)   For the purchase of appropriate dosimetry and QA/QC equipment necessary for commissioning and ongoing QA?

F.   Establishment of policies, procedures and protocols

(1)   Are policies and procedures in place?
  (i)   For radiation safety?
  (ii)   For emergency situations such as a ^{60}Co source that is stuck in the 'On' position?
  (iii)   For all clinical protocols?

(2)   Is there a plan in place for the acceptance and commissioning of the newly installed technology?
  (i)   Does the plan include well-defined timelines?

(3)   Are there documented QA protocols, policies and procedures?

(4)   Have clinical protocols been developed [42, 52, 57]?

(5)   Have imaging protocols been developed?

Appendix III

STANDARD EQUIPMENT PACKAGE FOR A RADIOTHERAPY DEPARTMENT

The procurement of an integrated radiotherapy equipment package is advisable for a standard radiotherapy clinic. The package can be adjusted depending on the individual requirements of each department.

III.1. UPGRADE PATHS FOR RADIOTHERAPY EQUIPMENT AND SOFTWARE

The standard radiotherapy equipment package detailed in Table 8 ideally includes all or some of the following upgrade paths as optional/future purchasable items:

(a) Record and verify systems (RVSs) were initially developed to reduce the risk of treatment errors, where the treatment parameters used for a given fraction were set manually and could differ from the 'prescribed' (or 'intended') parameters, leading to improved safety and improved efficiency [53]. Basic RVSs simply record and verify the radiotherapy treatment set-up, so they could be standalone systems. Advanced RVSs function as a wider intranet and provide an integral link in the planning, imaging, delivery and record-keeping processes.

(b) Electronic portal imaging devices (EPIDs) were first used to replace portal imaging with radiographic films, but digital images can be exploited further, in particular the possibility of on-line verification, remote review and dosimetry. A high quality imaging, low dose EPID, based on amorphous-silicon flat panel technology, is available, either as an integral upgradable part of the teletherapy unit or as an add-on system.

(c) A multileaf collimator (MLC) for the teletherapy unit facilitates the shaping of radiotherapy beams for the delivery of 3-D CRT and provides non-uniform fluence for IMRT treatments. If a teletherapy unit is equipped with an MLC, an RVS is required. Implementation of IMRT may require additional licences for treatment planning, the RVS and the treatment unit.

Both hardware and software components of these systems will be included. Furthermore, it needs to be emphasized that a lack of proper QC procedures for these systems may result in severe accidents from inaccurate information. Training of staff and extra staff also needs to be considered when the complexity of the radiotherapy service increases.

TABLE 8. STANDARD EQUIPMENT PACKAGE FOR A RADIOTHERAPY DEPARTMENT

Component	Equipment	Accessories	Comments
Teletherapy	Two matched units: 100 cm and 80 cm SAD[a] Co-60 units or standard single energy linacs	— Immobilization equipment, positioning lasers, CCTV[b] and intercommunication device — EPID[c] or port film equipment — Additional safety and security systems are required for Co-60	— Better to plan for two units, but may start with one unit — Consider land and architectural plans with generic MV bunkers — If the unit does not have an MLC[d] then the package includes an upgrade plan for both the TPS[e] and RVS[f]

TABLE 8. STANDARD EQUIPMENT PACKAGE FOR A RADIOTHERAPY DEPARTMENT (cont.)

Component	Equipment	Accessories	Comments
Simulation	Conventional simulator	Immobilization equipment, positioning lasers, output devices (e.g. printers)	
	CT[g] simulator or access to a diagnostic CT scanner	Immobilization equipment, positioning lasers, flat-top couch using the same indexing system as the treatment machine	The CT will be networked to the TPS
Treatment planning	3-D TPS	Mould room equipment	Some mould room equipment may not be necessary if both teletherapy units include MLC
Brachytherapy	Ir-192 or Co-60 HDR[h] brachytherapy unit, TPS/C-arm X ray device	Treatment couch, range of applicators, safety systems, CCTV and intercommunication device	In countries where gynaecological cancers are prevalent, brachytherapy treatment is usually the recommended treatment modality. Depending on the clinical indications, it can be delivered as monotherapy or as a boost to the external beam treatment
Teletherapy	Superficial/ orthovoltage X ray unit	Treatment couch, immobilization equipment, shielding, CCTV and intercommunication device	Access to electrons may replace orthovoltage based on local situation and epidemiology data, as well as major cancer sites
Dosimetry	Dosimetry and QA[i] equipment	Phantoms, calibrated dosimeters and ionization chambers, QC[j] and radiation protection, including personnel radiation monitoring equipment	Equipment adapted according to teletherapy unit. In vivo dosimetry will be considered according to national regulations
Training	Applications/ operational training		

[a] SAD: source to axis distance.
[b] CCTV: closed circuit television.
[c] EPID: electronic portal imaging device.
[d] MLC: multileaf collimator.
[e] TPS: treatment planning system.
[f] RVS: record and verify system.
[g] CT: computed tomography.
[h] HDR: high dose rate.
[i] QA: quality assurance.
[j] QC: quality control.

Appendix IV

CALCULATION OF THE NUMBER OF TREATMENT MACHINES

Starting from the number (No.) of treatment fractions (fr) on a machine per year and the average (av.) number of fractions per treatment course, Eq. (1) can help to determine the number of patients that can be treated per machine per year:

$$\left(\frac{\text{No. treated patients per machine}}{\text{year}} \right) = \left(\frac{\text{Annual No. fr per machine}}{\text{Av. No. fr per course of treatment}} \right) \tag{1}$$

where the annual number of treatment fractions that are delivered on a machine per year can be calculated according to Eq. (2):

$$\text{Annual No. fr per machine} = \left(\frac{\text{Av. No. fr}}{\text{hour}} \right) \times \left(\frac{\text{Treatment hours}}{\text{day}} \right) \times \left(\frac{\text{Treatment days}}{\text{year}} \right) \tag{2}$$

Note that the number of treatment days per year needs to take into account the number of unavailable days due to statutory holidays, as well as the number of days that are used for scheduled preventative maintenance, QA and expected downtime.

Once the number of treated patients per machine per year has been determined, the required number of machines can be calculated from the knowledge of the number of patients that are to be treated by the department, as shown in Appendix V.

Appendix V

EXAMPLE ILLUSTRATING THE METHOD SHOWN IN APPENDIX IV

V.1. CALCULATING THE NUMBER OF TREATMENT MACHINES

V.1.1. Determining the parameters

The parameters required for performing the calculation for the determination of numbers of machines include:

(a) Total number of patients to be treated per year;
(b) Average number of treatment fractions per patient;
(c) Total number of treatment fractions per year;
(d) Number of operational hours per day;
(e) Number of treatment days per year;
(f) Number of treatment fractions per hour.

Each of these is now addressed in more detail.

(a) Total number of patients to be treated per year

The total number of patients to be treated per year is dependent on the total population for the region from which the cancer patients are to receive treatment, the cancer incidence rate for that population and the radiotherapy utilization rate, as shown in Eq. (3):

$$\frac{\text{Total No. RT patients}}{\text{year}} = \text{Population base for radiotherapy facilities} \times \text{CI} \times \text{RTU} \qquad (3)$$

where RT is radiotherapy, CI is the cancer incidence and RTU is the radiotherapy utilization rate (i.e. the fraction of cancer patients requiring radiotherapy).

The total number of patients to be treated per year is dependent on the project that is being planned. If the total population from which all the cancer patients are to be treated is known, this is the number to be used. This could be for a specific region, or for an entire country. If it is for an entire country, the total population of that country is used. For this sample calculation, an LMIC in Africa with a population of 35 million people is assumed.

Cancer incidence data can be found from the national cancer control plan. If this is not available, detailed data can be found from GLOBOCAN [21]. Examples are shown in Fig. 3 and Table 9 for the top ten cancers in the specified African country.

Knowing which types of cancer are predominant, the number of fractions can be determined using radiotherapy utilization rates (RTU) (i.e. the fraction of cancer cases benefiting from radiotherapy) as described in a previous IAEA publication [17]. More recent RTUs for high income contexts can be found in Ref. [59].

Due to the variation in cancer types in different countries and world regions, the RTUs will also vary by region. The regional RTUs calculated by Zubizarreta et al. [62] are 0.543 for Africa, 0.533 for Latin America, 0.501 for Europe-Central Asia and 0.495 for Asia-Pacific. Thus, for this hypothetical LMIC, of the 23 170 total cancer cases listed in Table 9, 0.543 × 23 170 = 12 581 people will need radiotherapy.

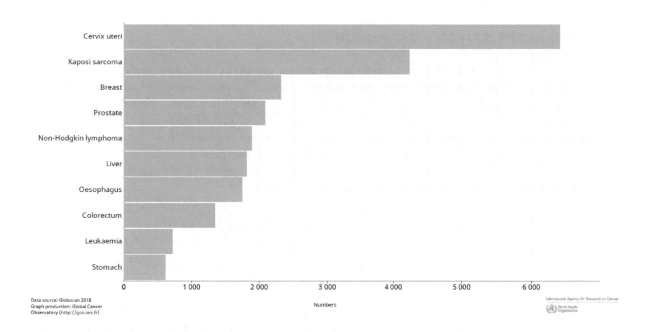

Data source: Globocan 2018
Graph production: Global Cancer
Observatory (http://gco.iarc.fr)

Numbers

International Agency for Research on Cancer
World Health Organization

FIG. 3. Example of a bar graph obtained from Cancer Today showing estimated incident data for the top ten cancers for both sexes in a specified country in Africa in 2018. Data source (2018): GLOBOCAN [21]. Graph production: Cancer Today (https://gco.iarc.fr/today/home).

TABLE 9. EXAMPLE OF A TABLE SHOWING ESTIMATED INCIDENT DATA FOR THE TOP TEN CANCERS FOR BOTH SEXES IN A SPECIFIED COUNTRY IN AFRICA IN 2018

(derived from Fig. 3 data sourced in 2018 from GLOBOCAN [21])

Cancer	Incidence
Cervix uteri	6 413
Kaposi sarcoma	4 238
Breast	2 318
Prostate	2 086
Non-Hodgkin lymphoma	1 888
Liver	1 811
Oesophagus	1 749
Colorectum	1 345
Leukaemia	711
Stomach	611
Total	23 170

(b)   Average number of treatment fractions per patient

The average number of treatment fractions per patient can be calculated by performing a detailed analysis of cancer types and numbers of fractions prescribed for each cancer type, and calculating a weighted average based on the cancer incidence. However, a simplified approach has been provided by Zubizarreta et al. [62], which also incorporates a retreatment rate of 25% with 3.3 fractions per retreatment course. The calculated number of average fractions per course is 16.44 for Africa, 16.53 for Latin America, 15.95 for Europe-Central Asia and 16.29 for Asia-Pacific.

(c)   Total number of treatment fractions per year

Based on the above data, the total number of treatment fractions per year is:

$$12\ 581 \times 16.44 = 206\ 836$$

Another source of information on the estimated number of fractions per country can be found in the supplementary data associated with the work of the 2015 Lancet Oncology Commission report [1]. The data include the estimated number of fractions per country for 2012, as well as projections out to 2035. For this example, it is assumed that this hypothetical country needs to treat 210 000 fractions based on the 2018 GLOBOCAN data [21]. Using the projection data of the supplementary data of Ref. [1], this would increase to about 504 000 fractions by the year 2035. For simplicity, a linear interpolation can be used to generate the appropriate data for the specific year of interest. Assuming planning for 2022, the estimated number of fractions is 297 000 per year.

(d)   Number of operational hours per day

The number of treatment hours per day is a decision that needs to be made based on local circumstances. Zubizarreta et al. [62] use two benchmarks, 8 hours per day and 10 hours per day. The Lancet Oncology Commission report [1] assumed 12 hours per day for its calculations and 16 hours per day for its 'efficiency' modelling. For this sample calculation, 10 hours per day are assumed.

(e)   Number of treatment days per year

The number of treatment days per year considers the number of statutory holidays per year. Typically, radiotherapy clinics operate 5 days per week. A given country or region will have a specified number of statutory holidays. For this sample calculation, 12 statutory holidays per year are assumed, giving $(52 \times 5) - 12 = 248$ treatment days per year.

(f)   Number of treatment fractions per hour

The Lancet Oncology Commission report [1] assumed 4 fractions per hour for its general estimations of 3-D CRT and 5 fractions per hour for its 'efficiency' modelling. In this sample calculation, 4 treatment fractions per hour for a 10 hour day are assumed.

V.1.2. Calculating machine fractions and numbers

(1)   Number of patient treatments per year per machine

Using Eq. (2) and the parameter data, the number of patient treatments per year per machine can be calculated:

$$\text{Annual No. fr per machine} = \left(\frac{\text{Av. No. fr}}{\text{hour}}\right) \times \left(\frac{\text{Treatment hours}}{\text{day}}\right) \times \left(\frac{\text{Treatment days}}{\text{year}}\right)$$
$$= 4 \times 10 \times 248$$
$$= 9920$$

(2)   Number of machines required

Using the data from Eq. (2), it is possible to calculate the number of machines required. For 297 000 fractions, 297 000/9 920 = 30 machines would be required. The total number of new machines required would have to be adjusted accordingly if existing departments already have machines.

V.2. ADDITIONAL CONSIDERATIONS

Several general comments need to be considered in relation to machine numbers.

V.2.1.   Complexity

The complexity of the treatment used impacts on the required number of machines. The assumption in this sample calculation is that 3-D CRT is used. If a substantial number of patients are going to be treated with IMRT and IGRT, patient throughput might reduce, for example, to as low as 2.5 patients per hour. If half of the patients are treated at the rate of 2.5 patients per hour and the other half at 4 patients per hour, 8060 fractions could be treated per year in a 10 hour day, which is effectively a 19% reduction in available treatment fractions compared to 3-D CRT. Alternatively, if 60–70% of the patients are palliative, patient throughput could possibly increase to 5–6 patients per hour with a corresponding increase in total number of patients treated per year.

V.2.2.   Training

The importance of appropriate training for all three major professions (medical physicists, radiation oncologists and RTTs) cannot be overstated. Planning for new and complex technologies without appropriate training can lead to significant problems. The IAEA publication on transitioning from 2-D to 3-D CRT to IMRT gives a more detailed description of what factors are to be considered [52].

V.2.3.   Special techniques

If the new or upgraded radiotherapy facility is considering the use of specialized techniques, these are considered in the planning process. Some techniques take a considerable amount of time and will reduce the available number of treatment fractions. Others may have an impact on room design and need careful consideration prior to room construction.

REFERENCES

[1] ATUN, R., et al., Expanding global access to radiotherapy, Lancet Oncol. **16** (2015) 1153–1186.

[2] YAP, M.L., et al., The benefits of providing external beam radiotherapy in low- and middle-income countries, Clin. Oncol. (R. Coll. Radiol.) **29** (2017) 72–83.

[3] PAGE, B.R., et al., Cobalt, linac, or other: What is the best solution for radiation therapy in developing countries? Int. J. Radiat. Oncol. Biol. Phys. **89** (2014) 476–480.

[4] SUIT, H.D., What's the optimum choice?, Int. J. Radiat. Oncol. Biol. Phys. **12** (1986) 1711–1712.

[5] SUSHEELA, S.P., REVANNASIDDAIAH, S., Rekindling the immortal debate — telecobalt versus linear accelerator, J. Cancer Res. Ther. **11** (2015) 243–244.

[6] INTERNATIONAL ATOMIC ENERGY AGENCY, Radiation Dose in Radiotherapy from Prescription to Delivery, IAEA-TECDOC-896, IAEA, Vienna (1996).

[7] MUNSHI, A., et al., Impact of adjuvant radiation therapy photon energy on quality of life after breast conservation therapy: Linear accelerator versus the cobalt machine, J. Cancer Res. Ther. **8** (2012) 361–366.

[8] VAN DER GIESSEN, P.H., Maintenance costs for cobalt machines and linear accelerators: new machines versus old, Radiother. Oncol. **62** (2002) 349–350.

[9] VAN DER GIESSEN, P.H., A comparison of maintenance costs of cobalt machines and linear accelerators, Radiother. Oncol. **20** (1991) 64–65.

[10] VAN DER GIESSEN, P.H., et al., Multinational assessment of some operational costs of teletherapy, Radiother. Oncol. **71** (2004) 347–355.

[11] RAVICHANDRAN, R., Has the time come for doing away with Cobalt-60 teletherapy for cancer treatments, J. Med. Phys. **34** (2009) 63–65.

[12] HEALY, B.J., VAN DER MERWE, D., CHRISTAKI, K.E., MEGHZIFENE, A., Cobalt-60 machines and medical linear accelerators: competing technologies for external beam radiotherapy, Clin. Oncol. (R. Coll. Radiol.) **29** (2017) 110–115.

[13] DATTA, N.R., SAMIEI, M., BODIS, S., Radiotherapy infrastructure and human resources in Europe — present status and its implications for 2020, Eur. J. Cancer **50** (2014) 2735–2743.

[14] BARTON, M.B., et al., Estimating the demand for radiotherapy from the evidence: a review of changes from 2003 to 2012, Radiother. Oncol. **112** (2014) 140–144.

[15] INTERNATIONAL ATOMIC ENERGY AGENCY, Setting Up a Radiotherapy Programme: Clinical, Medical Physics, Radiation Protection and Safety Aspects, IAEA, Vienna (2008).

[16] VAN DYK, J., BATTISTA, J., Cobalt-60: An old modality, a renewed challenge, Curr. Oncol. **3** (1996) 8–17.

[17] INTERNATIONAL ATOMIC ENERGY AGENCY, Planning National Radiotherapy Services: A Practical Tool, IAEA Human Health Series No. 14, IAEA, Vienna (2010).

[18] INTERNATIONAL ATOMIC ENERGY AGENCY, Dirac Database, IAEA, Vienna,
https://dirac.iaea.org

[19] VAN DYK, J., The Modern Technology of Radiation Oncology: A Compendium for Medical Physicists and Radiation Oncologists, Medical Physics Publishing, Madison, WI (1999).

[20] BROWN, D.W., et al., A framework for the implementation of new radiation therapy technologies and treatment techniques in low-income countries, Phys. Med. **30** (2014) 791–798.

[21] FERLAY, J., et al., Global Cancer Observatory: Cancer Today, International Agency for Research on Cancer, Lyon, France (2020),
https://gco.iarc.fr/today

[22] INTERNATIONAL ATOMIC ENERGY AGENCY, Radiotherapy Facilities: Master Planning and Concept Design Considerations, IAEA Human Health Reports No. 10, IAEA, Vienna (2014).

[23] JOINER, M., VAN DER KOGEL, A., Basic Clinical Radiobiology, 4th edn, CRC, Boca Raton, FL (2009).

[24] URTASUN, R.C., Does improved depth dose characteristics and treatment planning correlate with a gain in therapeutic results? Evidence from past clinical experience using conventional radiation sources, Int. J. Radiat. Oncol. Biol. Phys. **22** (1992) 235–239.

[25] FOOTE, R.L., et al., Radiation therapy for glottic cancer using 6-MV photons, Cancer **77** (1996) 381–386.

[26] FORTIN, A., ALLARD, J., ALBERT, M., ROY, J., Outcome of patients treated with cobalt and 6 MV in head and neck cancers, Head Neck **23** (2001) 181–188.

[27] VAN DYK, J., GALVIN, J.M., GLASGOW, G.P., PODGORSAK, E., The Physical Aspects of Total and Half Body Photon Irradiation: A Report of Task Group 29, Radiation Therapy Committee, Association of Physicists in Medicine, AAPM Report No. 17, AAPM, New York (1986).

[28] VAN DYK, J., Dosimetry for total body irradiation, Radiother. Oncol. 9 (1987) 107–118.

[29] MISZCZYK, L., TUKIENDORF, A., GABOREK, A., WYDMANSKI, J., An evaluation of half-body irradiation in the treatment of widespread, painful metastatic bone disease, Tumori 94 (2008) 813–821.

[30] MADANI, I., et al., Comparison of 6 MV and 18 MV photons for IMRT treatment of lung cancer, Radiother. Oncol. 82 (2007) 63–69.

[31] LAUGHLIN, J.S., MOHAN, R., KUTCHER, G.J., Choice of optimum megavoltage for accelerators for photon beam treatment, Int. J. Radiat. Oncol. Biol. Phys. 12 (1986) 1551–1557.

[32] STANTON, R., Dosimetric considerations in the choice of photon energy for external beam radiation therapy: Clinical examples, Med. Dosim. 16 (1991) 213–219.

[33] TYAGI, A., SUPE, S.S., SANDEEP, SINGH, M.P., A dosimetric analysis of 6 MV versus 15 MV photon energy plans for intensity modulated radiation therapy (IMRT) of carcinoma of cervix, Rep. Pract. Oncol. Radiother. 15 (2010) 125–131.

[34] YADAV, G., et al., Dosimetric influence of photon beam energy and number of arcs on volumetric modulated arc therapy in carcinoma cervix: A planning study, Rep. Pract. Oncol. Radiother. 22 (2017) 1–9.

[35] INTERNATIONAL ATOMIC ENERGY AGENCY, Radiation Oncology Physics: A Handbook for Teachers and Students, IAEA, Vienna (2005).

[36] INTERNATIONAL ATOMIC ENERGY AGENCY, Dosimetry of Small Static Fields Used in External Beam Radiotherapy, An International Code of Practice for Reference and Relative Dose Determination, IAEA Technical Reports Series No. 483, IAEA, Vienna (2017).

[37] INTERNATIONAL COMMISSION ON RADIATION UNITS AND MEASUREMENTS, Prescribing, Recording, and Reporting Intensity-Modulated Photon-Beam Therapy (IMRT), ICRU Rep. 83, ICRU, Oxford (2010).

[38] ADAMS, E.J., WARRINGTON, A.P., A comparison between cobalt and linear accelerator-based treatment plans for conformal and intensity-modulated radiotherapy, Br. J. Radiol. 81 (2008) 304–310.

[39] MACKIE, T.R., et al., Tomotherapy: A new concept for the delivery of dynamic conformal radiotherapy, Med. Phys. 20 (1993) 1709–1719.

[40] LANGHANS, M., et al., Development, physical properties and clinical applicability of a mechanical multileaf collimator for the use in Cobalt-60 radiotherapy, Phys. Med. Biol. 60 (2015) 3375–3387.

[41] WOOTEN, H.O., et al., Quality of intensity modulated radiation therapy treatment plans using a Co-60 magnetic resonance image guidance radiation therapy system, Int. J. Radiat. Oncol. 92 (2015) 771–778.

[42] INTERNATIONAL ATOMIC ENERGY AGENCY, Introduction of Image Guided Radiotherapy into Clinical Practice, IAEA Human Health Reports No. 16, IAEA, Vienna (2019).

[43] DAWSON, D.J., WISSING, W.W., TONKS, R.E., A doorless entry system for high-energy radiation therapy rooms, Med. Phys. 25 (1998) 199–201.

[44] GLASGOW, G.P., CORRIGAN, K.W., Installation of 60Co 100 cm source-to-axis distance teletherapy units in vaults designed for 80-cm units, Health Phys. 68 (1995) 411–415.

[45] REICHENVATER, H., MATIAS, L.D., Is Africa a 'graveyard' for linear accelerators? Clin. Oncol. (R. Coll. Radiol.) 28 (2016) e179–e183.

[46] DUROSINMI-ETTI, F.A., An overview of cancer management by radiotherapy in anglophone West Africa, Int. J. Radiat. Oncol. Biol. Phys. 19 (1990) 1263–1266.

[47] EUROPEAN COMMISSION, FOOD AND AGRICULTURE ORGANIZATION OF THE UNITED NATIONS, INTERNATIONAL ATOMIC ENERGY AGENCY, INTERNATIONAL LABOUR ORGANIZATION, OECD NUCLEAR ENERGY AGENCY, PAN AMERICAN HEALTH ORGANIZATION, UNITED NATIONS ENVIRONMENT PROGRAMME, WORLD HEALTH ORGANIZATION, Radiation Protection and Safety of Radiation Sources: International Basic Safety Standards, IAEA Safety Standards Series No. GSR Part 3, IAEA, Vienna (2014).

[48] INTERNATIONAL ATOMIC ENERGY AGENCY, INTERNATIONAL LABOUR OFFICE, PAN AMERICAN HEALTH ORGANIZATION, WORLD HEALTH ORGANIZATION, Radiation Protection and Safety in Medical Uses of Ionizing Radiation, IAEA Safety Standards Series No. SSG-46, IAEA, Vienna (2018).

[49] INTERNATIONAL ATOMIC ENERGY AGENCY, Lessons Learned from Accidental Exposures in Radiotherapy, IAEA Safety Reports Series No. 17, IAEA, Vienna (2000).

[50] INTERNATIONAL COMMISSION ON RADIOLOGICAL PROTECTION, Preventing accidental exposures from new external beam radiation therapy technologies, ICRP Publication No. 112, Ann. ICRP 39 (2009) 4.

[51] INTERNATIONAL ATOMIC ENERGY AGENCY, Staffing in Radiotherapy: An Activity Based Approach, IAEA Human Health Reports (CD-ROM) No. 13, IAEA, Vienna (2015).

[52] INTERNATIONAL ATOMIC ENERGY AGENCY, Transition from 2-D Radiotherapy to 3-D Conformal and Intensity Modulated Radiotherapy, IAEA-TECDOC-1588, IAEA, Vienna (2008).

[53] INTERNATIONAL ATOMIC ENERGY AGENCY, Record and Verify Systems for Radiation Treatment of Cancer: Acceptance Testing, Commissioning and Quality Control, IAEA Human Health Reports No. 7, IAEA, Vienna (2013).

[54] VAN DYK, J., ZUBIZARRETA, E., LIEVENS, Y., Cost evaluation to optimise radiation therapy implementation in different income settings: A time-driven activity-based analysis, Radiother. Oncol. **125** (2017) 178–185.

[55] INTERNATIONAL ATOMIC ENERGY AGENCY, IAEA Human Health Campus: Radiation Oncology, IAEA, Vienna,
https://humanhealth.iaea.org/HHW/RadiationOncology/index.html

[56] ZUBIZARRETA, E., VAN DYK, J., LIEVENS, Y., Analysis of global radiotherapy needs and costs by geographic region and income level, Clin. Oncol. (R. Coll. Radiol.) **29** (2017) 84–92.

[57] NILSSON, P., et al., A template for writing radiotherapy protocols, Acta Oncol. **54** (2015) 275–279.

[58] WORLD HEALTH ORGANIZATION, INTERNATIONAL ATOMIC ENERGY AGENCY, Technical Specifications of Radiotherapy Equipment for Cancer Treatment, WHO, Geneva (2021).

[59] WONG, K., DELANEY, G.P., BARTON, M.B., Evidence-based optimal number of radiotherapy fractions for cancer: A useful tool to estimate radiotherapy demand, Radiother. Oncol. **119** (2016) 145–149.

[60] ROSENBLATT, E., et al., Radiotherapy utilization in developing countries: An IAEA study, Radiother. Oncol. **128** (2018) 400–405.

[61] INTERNATIONAL ATOMIC ENERGY AGENCY, Security of Radioactive Material in Use and Storage and of Associated Facilities, IAEA Nuclear Security Series No. 11-G (Rev. 1), IAEA, Vienna (2019).

[62] ZUBIZARRETA, E.H., FIDAROVA, E., HEALY, B., ROSENBLATT, E., Need for radiotherapy in low and middle income countries — the silent crisis continues, Clin. Oncol. (R. Coll. Radiol.) **27** (2015) 107–114.

ABBREVIATIONS

CRT	conformal radiotherapy
CT	computed tomography
EPID	electronic portal imaging device
FFF	flattening filter free
IGRT	image guided radiotherapy
IMRT	intensity modulated radiotherapy
IT	information technology
LMIC	low and middle income country
MLC	multileaf collimator
RTT	radiation therapist
RTU	radiotherapy utilization rate
RVS	record and verify system
SAD	source to axis distance
TPS	treatment planning system
VMAT	volumetric arc therapy

CONTRIBUTORS TO DRAFTING AND REVIEW

Agarwal, J.P.	Tata Memorial Hospital, India
Carrara, M.	International Atomic Energy Agency
Cheung, Kin Yin	Prince of Wales Hospital, Hong Kong, China
Christaki, K.	International Atomic Energy Agency
Deshpande, D.	Tata Memorial Hospital, India
Esteban Sanz, D.	Nuclear Medicine School Foundation, Argentina
Gershkevitch, E.	North Estonia Medical Centre Foundation, Estonia
Gilley, D.	International Atomic Energy Agency
Gondhowiardjo, S.	Cipto Mangunkusumo General Hospital, Indonesia
Kennedy, J.W.P.	Cochrane, Canada
Meghzifene, A.	International Atomic Energy Agency
van der Merwe, D.	International Atomic Energy Agency
Van Dyk, J.	Western University, Canada
Zubizarreta, E.	International Atomic Energy Agency

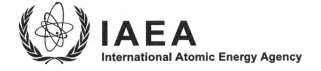

ORDERING LOCALLY

IAEA priced publications may be purchased from the sources listed below or from major local booksellers.

Orders for unpriced publications should be made directly to the IAEA. The contact details are given at the end of this list.

NORTH AMERICA

Bernan / Rowman & Littlefield

15250 NBN Way, Blue Ridge Summit, PA 17214, USA

Telephone: +1 800 462 6420 • Fax: +1 800 338 4550

Email: orders@rowman.com • Web site: www.rowman.com/bernan

REST OF WORLD

Please contact your preferred local supplier, or our lead distributor:

Eurospan Group

Gray's Inn House

127 Clerkenwell Road

London EC1R 5DB

United Kingdom

Trade orders and enquiries:

Telephone: +44 (0)176 760 4972 • Fax: +44 (0)176 760 1640

Email: eurospan@turpin-distribution.com

Individual orders:

www.eurospanbookstore.com/iaea

For further information:

Telephone: +44 (0)207 240 0856 • Fax: +44 (0)207 379 0609

Email: info@eurospangroup.com • Web site: www.eurospangroup.com

Orders for both priced and unpriced publications may be addressed directly to:

Marketing and Sales Unit

International Atomic Energy Agency

Vienna International Centre, PO Box 100, 1400 Vienna, Austria

Telephone: +43 1 2600 22529 or 22530 • Fax: +43 1 26007 22529

Email: sales.publications@iaea.org • Web site: www.iaea.org/publications